LCHF
Low Carb High Fat

Diet & Cookbook

Your Guide and Recipes

for Weight Loss and Healthy Living

WaraWaran Roongruangsri

Pawana Publishing

Good Health Content

Low Carb High Fat Diet & Cookbook

Copyright © 2016 WaraWaran Roongruangsri

All rights reserved.

Low Carb High Fat Diet & Cookbook

> *"One cannot think well, love well, sleep well,
> if one has not dined well."*
> *-Virginia Woolf*

First Publish in 2016 by Pawana Publishing
Copyright © 2016 WaraWaran Roongruangsri
Pawana © is a registered trademark of Pawana Publishing.
Cover and interior design by Pawana Publishing
Interior photos © Pawana Publishing
Author photo by Pawana Publishing

All rights reserved.

No part of this publication may be reproduced or distribute in any form or by means, electronic or mechanical, or stored in database or retrieval system without prior written from the publisher.

ISBN-13: 978-1523610297
ISBN-10: 1523610298

This document is geared towards providing exact and reliable information in regards to the topic and issue covered. The publication is sold with the idea that the publisher is not required to render accounting, officially permitted, or otherwise, qualified services. If advice is necessary, legal or professional, a practiced individual in the profession should be ordered.

- From a Declaration of Principles which was accepted and approved equally by a Committee of the American Bar Association and a Committee of Publishers and Associations.

In no way is it legal to reproduce, duplicate, or transmit any part of this document in either electronic means or in printed format. Recording of this publication is strictly prohibited and any storage of this document is not allowed unless with written permission from the publisher. All rights reserved.

The information provided herein is stated to be truthful and consistent, in that any liability, in terms of inattention or otherwise, by any usage or abuse of any policies, processes, or directions contained within is the solitary and utter responsibility of the recipient reader. Under no circumstances will any legal responsibility or blame be held against the publisher for any reparation, damages, or monetary loss due to the information herein, either directly or indirectly.

Respective authors own all copyrights not held by the publisher.

The information herein is offered for informational purposes solely, and is universal as so. The presentation of the information is without contract or any type of guarantee assurance.

The trademarks that are used are without any consent, and the publication of the trademark is without permission or backing by the trademark owner. All trademarks and brands within this book are for clarifying purposes only and are the owned by the owners themselves, not affiliated with this document.

Author's Note

Finding a diet plan that works for you can be confusing and frustrating. There are so many that are out there and all of them claim that they are better than the others and will provide you with the best results. With all of the options that are out there, how do you choose the one that works for you?

If you've tried out many different weight loss and diet plans, you may be tired of working hard and not seeing the results that you desire. For those that feel like they're stuck in a rut, the Low Carb High Fat diet may be the answer that you need. Instead of getting on another diet plan that sounds like all of the others and is difficult to maintain, the LCHF diet plan will give you simple, easy to follow steps that will help you to drop the weight while still feeling full and satisfied. The best part is, that if you are able to follow some of the basic requirements of this diet plan, then you will not have to waste your time with counting calories or weighing food in order to lose the weight!

This book "LCHF: Low Carb High Fat Diet & Cookbook, Your Guide and Recipes for Weight Loss and Healthy Living" will provide you with the information that you need in order to get started and be successful on the LCHF diet. You'll find chapters with information on topics such as:

- What is the Low Carb High Fat Diet?
- LCHF for Beginners
- How the LCHF Works
- Foods to eat and foods to avoid on the LCHF diet
- Recipes for breakfast, lunch, dinner, as well as desserts and snacks

Learn how easy it can be to lose weight without the extra work required by other diet plans by checking out this guidebook today!

Thanks for downloading this book. I hope you enjoy reading it!

WaraWaran Roongruangsri

Low Carb High Fat Diet & Cookbook

CONTENTS

Author's Note	iii
1. LCHF Introduction	1
2. LCHF for Beginners	10
3. How the LCHF Works	12
4. What to Eat for LCHF	18
5. LCHF Breakfasts Recipes	20
6. LCHF Lunch and Dinner Recipes	25
7. LCHF Snacks and Desserts	35

"Tell me what you eat, and I will tell you who you are."

- Brillat-Savarin

1. LCHF Introduction

For years, we've been told to fear fat. Filling your plate with the "F" word has been seen as an express ticket to heart disease. Low-carb, high-fat diets, like Atkins, were ridiculed for causing high cholesterol while giving followers a license to gorge on damaging red meats and full-fat cheeses. Meanwhile, carb-loading became popular with endurance athletes as a way to avoid the feared hitting-of-the-wall.

Then, trends began to change. Common criticism of the Atkins diet was debunked: Popular science suggested that a low-carb, high-fat diet actually *improved* HDL, or "good" cholesterol, and didn't worsen LDL, or "bad" cholesterol. In the 1980s, Stephen Phinney, an MIT medical researcher, noticed that the carb-loading math just didn't add up.

Our bodies only have a limited store of glycogen, which fuels your muscles, about 2,500 calories of carbs in reserve at all times—and this can be quickly depleted on long runs. But our bodies have about *50,000* calories of fat stored—a much deeper pool to pull from.

Phinney wondered if athletes could train their bodies to burn fat instead of carbs. Your body naturally burns carbs to keep your muscles moving—and carbs are the quickest form of fuel to convert into energy. But "think of glycogen as the gas in the tank of the car," says Pam Bede, R.D., sports dietitian for Abbott's EAS Sports Nutrition. When that gas is low, you need to refuel, which is where energy gels and GUs come in. If your body could burn fat, Phinney thought, you could go a heck of a lot longer before refueling.

So Phinney put a small group of elite male cyclists on a low-carb diet to test it out—forcing their bodies to tap into the fat stores. While plenty of studies show that a low-carb, high-fat diet results in *lower* peak power and VO2 max, meaning it generally makes you slower, he found that, indeed, cyclists performed just as well on a two and a half hour ride when they ate a diet low in carbs and high in fat as when they ate their traditional training diet.

And thus, the low-carb, high-fat (LCHF) diet was born. What is the LCHF? With an ideal meal plan, you're taking in roughly 50 percent of your calories from healthy fats, 25 from carbs, and 25 from protein. For comparison, the current government recommendation is 30 percent of calories from fat, 50 to 60 percent from carbs, and 10 to 20 from protein.

The problem? Phinney's model was imperfect: When he tested cyclist's sprinting capabilities on the LCHF diet, he noticed fat-fueled athletes clocked in at a slower time than normal. Fast forward some 40 years, though, and award-winning-triathletes like Simon Whitfield and Ben Greenfield have renounced the church of carbs in favor of a low-carb, high-fat diet. Recently, a reality star famously went low-carb to shed her baby weight. She attributed her impressive 45-pound weight loss to a similar eating plan.

But with mixed research and confusing star-studded testimonials—does the diet work? And, more importantly, is it healthy?

Can It Improve Your Fitness?
The effect of a low-carb, high-fat diet on athletic performance has only been looked at in a handful of studies since Phinney's original experiment. And when it comes to high speeds, Bede says it makes sense why a LCHF would slow you down: "Carbs are a fairly efficient way to burn fuel, so if you're running

at high speeds and need that energy immediately, carbohydrates are going to be a better source of fuel," Bede explains. But because it takes longer for your body to access the energy in fat, you won't be able to perform as quickly.

If you're focused on distance and not speed, though, don't write off the LCHF so soon. It can actually help with that moment every runner dreads: hitting the wall. "In endurance athletes, adapting as much as possible to use fat can help those who struggle with bonking. It can help delay that significant onset of fatigue, which is favorable because it enables an athlete to rely less on carbohydrate gels or fluid carbohydrates—and to go faster for longer," says Georgie Fear, R.D., author of *Lean Habits For Lifelong Weight Loss*. Another added bonus: You'll avoid the all-too-common side effect of gastric distress from race gels and GUs.

But like much of the LCHF research, the scientific evidence is mixed—it's still a vastly under-researched area. The most promising study to date is expected to come out later this year from Jeff Volek, Ph.D., R.D., at the Ohio State University, the second most prolific researcher on the topic next to Phinney.

Beyond the research, there's also a growing wave of triathletes and ultra-runners who attribute their success to jumping on the fat-fueling bandwagon. Fitness coach Ben Greenfield finished the 2013 Ironman Canada in under 10 hours while consuming almost no carbs, while ultra-runner Timothy Olson set a record for fastest completion of the Western States 100-mile course on a LCHF diet. "Athletes I work with say that once they got used to the diet, they feel better than they ever have before, their performance is potentially better, but certainly no worse, and they don't have sugar cravings or mood swings like when they were trying to fuel with carbs," Bede says.

Whether or not it improves performance, teaching your body to pull from your fat reserves, which you can do by simply switching to the diet, does offer better blood sugar stability. This helps to prevent hypoglycemia, or low blood sugar.

A new study in *Exercise and Sport Sciences Reviews has found that the* LCHF also helped strength athletes to lose fat without compromising their strength or power. That means that while people may not have seen performance gains, performance didn't suffer, plus they lost weight, Bede explains.

But Can the LCHF Really Help You Lose Weight?

While the now-popular weight loss angle has gotten slightly more scientific attention thanks to interested nutrition researchers, there is yet to be overwhelming evidence in either direction. But most of the limited research on weight loss and the LCHF has been in favor of it.

In theory, it makes sense that you'd lose weight: "Carbohydrates attract water, so part of the initial weight loss is shedding of water stores," says Bede. "More importantly, though, fat is very satiating. While it does have more calories per gram than a carbohydrate, you can only eat so much before you are full—similar to protein." With carbs, you can finish that whole bag of pretzels and still be hungry. If you're avoiding refined carbs, you're also avoiding the cravings for more unhealthy foods that research has shown they cause.

A study last year in the *Annals of Internal Medicine* made one of the most convincing cases yet: Researchers found that men and women who switched to a low-carb diet lost 14 pounds after one year—eight pounds more than those who limited their fat intake instead. The high-fat group also maintained more muscle, trimmed more body fat, and increased their protein intake more than their carb-heavy counterparts. These results are promising not only because researchers looked at the diet long-term, but also because they didn't limit how many calories the participants could eat, debunking the idea that the

LCHF only works as well as any other calorie-capped diet.

Should You Try the Diet?
No one agrees that the LCHF is perfect for everyone, or ideal for anyone for that matter. But whether you should even try it is up for debate among our experts. Fear, for example, isn't crazy about LCHF as a sustainable diet dogma. "I've just seen too many people end up sick, burned out, and feeling awful," she explains.

Conversely, Bede has seen it work for many of her athlete clients. And scientific evidence proves that there is little harm, other than to your speed, in trying it out. It'll likely help you lose weight, and there is still a chance it'll increase your distance or power performance.
And if your first response to hearing "restrict your carbs" is "yeah right," you don't actually have to be quite so rigid: The high-fat group in the *Annals of Internal Medicine* study made all of their weight-loss gains despite the fact that they never actually kept their carb goals as low as the study guidelines.

At its roots, the LCHF is all about healthy eating, which *everyone* can benefit from. "You're eating mostly fruits, vegetables, heart-healthy oils, with some full-fat dairy and a touch of whole grains, all of which are a recipe for optimal health," Bede says. And this brings up the point: "The benefit of the diet could potentially be in ditching the junk and loading up on the whole foods more than the actual fat itself."

Just be aware that you have to give your body at least two weeks to learn how to use fat as fuel, a phase known as fat adaptation, Bede advises. "If you're continuously feeling fatigued during your run from a LCHF diet after that, you may not be responding well to it." Ideally, you'd try the diet before training starts so the adjustment period doesn't affect your mileage or time goals, she adds.

How to Achieve 50 Percent Fat, 25 Percent Carbs, 25 Percent Protein

We discussed earlier how you skip refined carbs for whole grains in traditional diets. Well, your fats on a LCHF diet should come from healthy sources as well: full-fat dairy, nuts, and oils. And while saturated fats, like those in cheese, have gotten the biggest reputation makeover, there is still a place for unsaturated fats in your diet as well. The small amount of carbs that you eat on this diet will ideally come from produce. And, most importantly, you need to be eating enough protein.

2. LCHF for Beginners

A LCHF diet means you eat fewer carbohydrates and a higher intake of fat. Most importantly you minimize your intake of sugar and starches. Don't fear, there are many other delicious foods you can eat to feel satisfied and still lose weight.

A number of recent high-quality scientific studies shows that a LCHF makes it easier both to lose weight and to control your blood sugar. And that's just the beginning!

The basics
- **What to** Eat: Meat, fish, eggs, vegetables growing above ground and natural fats (like butter and coconut oil).

- What to Avoid: Sugar, starchy, and processed foods (like bread, pasta, rice, beans and potatoes).
- Eat when you're hungry, stop when you're satisfied. It's that simple.
- No need to count calories or weigh your food.
- Forget about industrially produced low fat products.

There are solid scientific reasons why LCHF works. When you avoid sugar and starches your blood sugar stabilizes and the levels of insulin, the fat-storing hormone, drop. This increases fat burning and makes you feel more satiated.

Note for diabetics

Avoiding the carbohydrates that raise your blood sugar decreases your need for medication to lower it. Taking the same dose of insulin as you did prior to adopting a low-carb diet might result in hypoglycemia (low blood sugar). You will likely need to test your blood sugar frequently when starting this diet and adapt (lower) your medication. This should be done with the assistance of a knowledgeable physician.

3. How the LCHF Works

What are you designed to eat?
Humans have evolved over millions of years as hunter-gatherers, without eating large amounts of carbohydrates. We ate the food available to us in nature by hunting, fishing and gathering all the edible foods we could find. These foods did not include pure starch in the form of bread, pasta, rice or potatoes. We have only eaten these starchy foods for 500-1,000 years, since the development of agriculture. Only a limited adaptation of our genes takes place in such a relatively short time.

100 - 200 years ago, with the Industrial Revolution, the concept of the factory was born and we were able to manufacture large amounts of pure sugar and white flour. Rapidly digested pure carbohydrates. We've

hardly had time to genetically adapt to these processed foods.

In the 1980s, the fear of fat gripped the western world. Low-fat products popped up on every shelf in the grocery store. The problem is, the less fat you eat, the more carbohydrates you need to feel satiated. And it's at this time in history that the disastrous epidemic of obesity and diabetes started. The most fat-phobic country in the world, the United States, was hit the hardest and is now the world's most obese country.

Today, it's become clear that the fear of real food with natural fat contents has been a big mistake.

The problem with sugar and starch
All digestible carbohydrates are broken down into simple sugars once they enter the intestines. The sugar is then absorbed into the blood, which raises the blood glucose levels. This then increases the production of the hormone insulin, our fat storing hormone.

Insulin is produced in the pancreas. In large amounts, it prevents fat from burning and stores surplus nutrients in fat cells. After a few hours or less, this can result in a perceived shortage of nutrients in the blood, creating feelings of hunger as well as cravings for something sweet. It is at that point that people will usually eat again. This starts the process once again: A vicious cycle leading to weight gain.

On the other hand, a low intake of carbs gives you a lower, more stable blood glucose, and lower amounts of insulin. This increases the release of fat from your fat stores and increases the fat burning. This usually leads to fat loss, especially around the belly in abdominally obese individuals.

Weight loss without hunger
The LCHF diet makes it easier for the body to use up its fat stores, as their release is no longer blocked by high insulin levels. This may be one reason why eating fat produces a feeling of longer-lasting satiety than carbohydrates. Numerous studies have shown: When people eat all they want on a low carb diet caloric intake typically drops.

So, no counting or food weighing is necessary. You can forget about the calories and trust your feelings of hunger and satiety. Most people don't need to count or weigh their food any more than they need to count their breathing. If you don´t believe it, just try for a couple of weeks and see for yourself!

Health as a bonus
No animal in nature need the assistance of nutritional expertise or calorie charts to eat. And still, as long as they eat the food they are designed to eat they stay at a normal weight and they avoid caries, diabetes and heart disease. Why would humans be an exception? Why would you be an exception?

In scientific studies not only has weight improved on a low carb diet, blood pressure, blood sugar and cholesterol profile (HDL, triglycerides) have also been improved. A calm stomach and less cravings for sweet food are also common experiences.

Initial side effects
If you stop eating sugar and starch cold turkey, which is recommended, you may experience some side effects as your body adjusts. For most people these side effects tend to be mild and last only a few days.

Common side effects in the first week:
- Headache
- Fatigue
- Dizziness
- Heart palpitations
- Irritability

The side effects will begin to rapidly subside as your body adapts and your fat burning increases. They can be minimized by drinking more fluids and by temporarily increasing your salt intake a bit. A good option is to drink some broth every few hours. Alternatively, drink a few extra glasses of water and put a little extra salt on your food.

The reason for this is that carbohydrate-rich foods may increase the water retention in your body. When you stop eating high-carb foods you'll lose excess water through your kidneys. This can result in dehydration and a lack of salt during the first week, before the body has adapted.

To minimize the side effects, some people prefer to decrease their intake of carbohydrates slowly, over a few weeks. But the "Nike way" (Just Do It) is probably the best choice for most people. Removing most sugar and starch often results in several pounds lost on the scale within a few days. It'll likely be mostly fluids but it's great for motivation.

4. What to Eat for LCHF

Eat all you like
- **Meat:** Any type, including beef, pork, wild game (deer, duck, etc.), chicken, turkey, etc. Feel free to eat the fat on the meat as well as the skin on the chicken. If possible try to choose high-quality organic or grass fed meat.
- **Fish and shellfish:** All kinds: Fatty fish such as salmon, mackerel or herring are great. Avoid breading.
- **Eggs:** All kinds: Boiled, fried, omelettes, etc. Free range, organic eggs are best.
- **Natural fat, high-fat sauces:** Using butter and cream for cooking can make your food taste better and make you feel more satiated. Try a Béarnaise or Hollandaise sauce, check the ingredients or, even better, make it

yourself. Coconut oil and olive oil are also good options.
- **Vegetables that grow above ground:** All kinds of cabbage, such as cauliflower, broccoli, cabbage and Brussels sprouts. Asparagus, zucchini, eggplant, olives, spinach, mushrooms, cucumber, lettuce, avocado, onions, peppers, tomatoes etc.
- **Dairy products:** Always select full-fat options like real butter, cream (40% fat), sour cream, Greek/Turkish yogurt and high-fat cheeses. Be careful with regular milk and skim milk as they contain a lot of lactose (milk sugar). Avoid flavored, sugary and low-fat dairy products.
- **Nuts:** A great alternative to candy, when snacking in front of the TV. Be sure to eat in moderation.
- **Berries:** Okay in moderation, if you are not a super strict or sensitive. Wonderful with fresh whipped cream.

What to Avoid
- **Sugar:** The worst. Soft drinks, candy, juice, sports drinks, chocolate, cakes, buns, pastries, ice cream, breakfast cereals. Preferably avoid sweeteners such as honey, syrups, and jellies as well.

- **Starch:** Bread, pasta, rice, potatoes, French fries, potato chips, porridge, muesli and so on. Wholegrain products are just less bad. Legumes, such as beans and lentils, are high in carbs. Moderate amounts of root vegetables (carrots, parsnips, beets, etc.) may be OK (unless you're eating extremely low carb).
- **Margarine:** Industrially imitated butter, with unnaturally high content of omega-6 fat, has no health benefits and tastes bad. It's been statistically linked to asthma, allergies and other inflammatory diseases.
- **Beer:** Liquid bread. Full of rapidly absorbed carbs, unfortunately.
- **Fruit:** Very sweet. Tropical fruits, in particular, contain lots of sugar. Only eat every once in a while. Treat fruit as a natural form of candy.

Once in a while

You decide when the time is right. Your weight loss may slow down a bit.

- **Alcohol:** Dry wine (regular red or dry white wine), whisky, brandy, vodka and cocktails without sugary mixers. Vodka and plain seltzer water with lime is a wise choice.
- **Dark chocolate:** Above 70% cocoa, keep portion size small.

Drink on most days

- **Water**

- **Coffee:** Try it with heavy cream.
- **Tea**

5. LCHF Breakfasts Recipes

Suggestions for low-carb breakfasts:
- Eggs and bacon
- Omelet
- Leftovers from last night's dinner
- Coffee with heavy cream
- A can of mackerel and hard boiled eggs
- Hard boiled egg with mayonnaise or cheese
- Avocado, salmon and sour cream
- Sandwich on low carb easy bread
- Cheese
- Boiled eggs mashed with butter, chopped chives, salt and pepper
- A piece of brie cheese and some ham or salami
- High-fat yogurt with nuts and seeds (and maybe berries)

Low-Carb Breakfasts Recipes

Scrambled Eggs with Basil
Ingredients, 1 serving
>2 eggs
>
>2 tablespoons coconut cream, yogurt or sour cream
>
>Salt
>
>Fresh basil
>
>Butter

Instructions
1. Melt butter in a pan on low heat. Mix together the eggs, coconut cream, salt and add to the pan. Stir with a spatula from the edge towards the center until the eggs are scrambled. For soft and creamy eggs, stir often on lower heat.
2. Serve with chopped, fresh basil.

Low Carb Easy Bread
6–8 pieces
Ingredients
>¼ cup (50 ml) sour cream
>
>2 egg whites
>
>2 teaspoons psyllium-seed husk (found in most health food stores)
>
>½ cup (100 ml) almond flour
>
>½ cup (100 ml) sesame seeds
>
>¼ cup (50 ml) sunflower seeds

1½ teaspoon baking powder
1 pinch salt

Instructions
1. Preheat oven to 400°F (200°C).
2. Whisk together egg whites and sour cream in a bowl.
3. Mix together the remaining ingredients and work in to the egg mixture. Let rest for a few minutes.
4. Form into rounds and place in a baking dish. Sprinkle some extra sesame seeds on top, if desired.
5. Bake in oven for 10–12 minutes.

LCHF Pancakes with Berries and Whipped Cream

2 servings

Ingredients

4 large eggs
1 cup (250 g) cottage cheese
2 tablespoons ground psyllium seed husk
2 tablespoons butter or coconut oil
Serve with
½–¾ cup (1–2 dl) fresh blueberries, raspberries or strawberries
full fat yogurt or fresh whipped cream

Instructions
1. Whisk the first three ingredients together until well combined. Let rest for at least 5 minutes.

2. Heat butter or oil in a frying pan and fry the pancakes on medium heat for 3–4 minutes on each side. Flip carefully.
3. Serve with berries and yogurt or whipped cream.

Avocado Eggs with Bacon Sails

This is a fun breakfast looks as good as it tastes and is appreciated by both young and old. A great recipe for the weekend, when you have a little bit more time in the morning.

Ingredients (per serving)

> 2 hard-boiled eggs
> ½ avocado
> ¼ package bacon
> Salt and pepper to taste

Instructions

1. Hard boil the eggs, let cool and split the eggs as if you were making deviled eggs.
2. Scoop out the yolk and mash with the avocado and salt and pepper to taste.
3. Bake the bacon until crispy in the oven for 5–7 minutes at 350°F (180°C) or in a frying pan.
4. Put the yolk mixture back into the egg and set the bacon sail!

Salad Sandwiches with Ideas for Fillings
Ingredients

It isn't impossible to have sandwiches without bread! Choose a lettuce variety that is crisp and firm, preferably romaine or leaf lettuce. Rinse the lettuce thoroughly and use as a carrier for the fillings. Suggested fillings:

- Cheese slices
- Avocado
- Dried meat
- Tomato
- Tuna salad
- Hard boiled eggs

The nutrient calculation is of course very approximate, depending on filling choices and amounts.

6. LCHF Lunch and Dinner Recipes

Chicken Alfredo à la Low-Carb, High-Fat
4 servings

Ingredients

Pasta
>4 large eggs
>6 egg yolks
>⅔ cup (200 ml) water
>2 tablespoons olive oil
>
>⅖ cups (100 ml) psyllium husk
>4 tablespoons coconut flour
>2½ teaspoons herb salt

Sauce
>2 lbs (1 kg) boneless chicken breasts
>⅔ lb fried bacon

1¼ cups (300 ml) heavy whipping cream
⅔ cup (200 ml) whole milk
⅔ cup (200 ml) parmesan cheese
4 garlic cloves
4 tablespoons pesto sauce
Salt, black pepper
8 fresh mushrooms, thinly sliced
1 large red bell pepper, thinly sliced
Butter to sauté in

Instructions

1. Preheat oven to 300°F (150°C). Start with the pasta: Whisk the eggs until fluffy, add water and olive oil.
2. Mix together the dry ingredients and whisk into the egg mixture Let rest for 7–8 minutes. Stir.
3. Spread the batter onto two sheets of parchment paper. Place plastic wrap on top and roll out towards the edges of the papers. Try to spread evenly and thinly. Alternatively, a pasta roller or machine can be used, if available.
4. Remove the plastic foil before baking. Bake for about 10 minutes. Let cool and remove the top paper and roll up from the short side. Then cut into strips with a sharp knife. Turn the oven temperature up to 400°F (200°C).
5. Clean the chicken breasts and split lengthwise so that you get two filets. Add salt and pepper and fry in butter at medium heat until the fillets are cooked through and golden brown. Place in a baking dish and bake in oven, about 10 minutes.

Fry the bacon until crisp. Shred the parmesan cheese. Bring the cream to a simmer, stir in finely chopped garlic and pesto and season with salt and pepper.
6. Sauté the sliced peppers and mushrooms in butter, season with salt and pepper. Mix the pasta with the vegetables and pour about half the sauce on top. Place the chicken on top of everything together with a couple of bacon strips and perhaps a little more parmesan cheese! Serve with remaining Alfredo sauce on the side.

Spinach and Goat-Cheese Pie
6 servings
Ingredients
Pie crust
> 1½ cups (3 dl) almond flour
> ¼ cup (½ dl) sesame seeds
> 1 tablespoon psyllium husk, ground
> ½ teaspoon salt
> 1.5 ounces (40 g) butter
> 1 egg

Egg batter
> 4-5 large eggs
> 1 cup (2-3 dl) heavy whipping cream or sour cream
> salt and pepper

Spinach and goat-cheese filling
> ½ pound (200 g) fresh spinach

2 tablespoons butter or coconut oil

1 clove of garlic

1 pinch ground nutmeg

salt and pepper

4 ounces (100 g) shredded cheese (cheddar or mozzarella work great)

6 ounces (150 g) goat cheese, sliced

Instructions

1. Mix almond flour and sesame seeds in a blender. Add the remaining ingredients and mix to form a dough. Press the dough into a springform pan and prick holes with a fork.
2. Whisk together the eggs with the heavy whipping cream or sour cream. Add salt and pepper. Add the filling in the following steps.
3. Chop the spinach coarsely. Finely chop the garlic. Brown the garlic in the butter or oil for a few minutes. Add the spinach and sauté until the spinach is wilted. Season with salt and pepper.
4. Add the chopped spinach to the pre-baked pie shell. Mix the grated cheese into the egg batter and pour over spinach. Top with goat cheese. Bake at 350°F (175°C) 30–40 minutes, until the egg are set in the middle of the pie.

Vegetarian LCHF Saturday: Halloumi Burger with Rutabaga Fries

Ingredients

 1 pound (400 g) halloumi cheese
 butter or coconut oil for frying
 4 large iceberg lettuce leaves
 1 tomato
 1 avocado
 ½ cup (1 dl) sour cream
 ½ cup (1 dl) mayonnaise
 ½ cup (1 dl) ajvar relish
 ½ rutabaga (swede, turnip)
 ½ cup (1 dl) coconut oil
 cheese bread, recipe below

Cheese bread:

 4 large eggs
 4 ounces (100 gram) cream cheese
 1.5 tablespoon ground psyllium husk
 2 teaspoons baking powder
 2 tablespoons chia seeds
 2 cups (5 dl) grated cheese
 topping: black poppy seeds + sea salt

Instructions

1. Preheat oven to 400°F (200°C)
2. Whisk eggs until fluffy, about 5 minutes
3. Mix in dry ingredients, and then blend the cream cheese into everything
4. Let rest for about 10 minutes
5. Put 8 large scoops of batter on a baking sheet and bake in the middle of the oven for 10–15 minutes

until they turn golden brown. Let cool before serving

Burger and fries:

1. Preheat oven to 450°F (225°C). Peel and cut the rutabaga into thin strips. Boil for 3-5 minutes in salted water. Let drain in a strainer.
2. Melt the coconut oil and toss with the rutabaga so that all strips are covered. Sprinkle with salt. Place strips on a baking sheet and bake until golden brown on the outside and soft on the inside. Turn once while baking. Rutabaga fries won't be as crispy as the potato fries as they don't contain as much starch but they taste great anyway.
3. For the dressing, mix the sour cream, mayonnaise, and ajvar relish together in a small bowl. Keep cool in the refrigerator.
4. Let rest for about 10 minutes
5. Assemble the burgers by placing rinsed lettuce, sliced tomato, and avocado onto the baked cheese bread. Quickly pan fry the helloumi cheese until it turns golden and add to the burger. Enjoy!

Bacon Mushroom Cheeseburger Lettuce Wraps

4 servings, about 12 lettuce wraps

Ingredients

- 12 slices of thick cut bacon
- 4 ounces (100 g) mushrooms, sliced
- 1½ lbs (680 g) ground beef
- ½ tsp salt
- ¼ tsp pepper
- 1 cup (240 ml) shredded cheddar cheese
- 1 small head iceberg lettuce, leaves separated and washed
- Additional salt and pepper to taste

Instructions

1. In a large skillet, cook bacon to desired crispness. Remove and let drain on a paper towel-lined plate.
2. Add the sliced mushrooms to the pan and sauté until browned and tender, about 5 to 7 minutes. Remove from pan and set aside.
3. Add the ground beef and season with salt and pepper. Sauté until beef is cooked through, about 10 minutes, breaking up chunks with the back of a wooden spoon.

4. Spoon ground beef into lettuce leaves, sprinkle with cheddar cheese and top with bacon and mushrooms.

Zucchini Patties with Tangy Tzatziki

4 servings
Ingredients

Zucchini patties:

2 zucchinis

1.5 tablespoon psyllium seed husk

4 large eggs

1 teaspoon onion powder

1/2 teaspoon paprika powder

salt and pepper

2 ounces (50 g) butter

Tzatziki:

½ cucumber, grated

1 cup (2 dl) Russian yogurt or sour cream

⅓ cup (¾ dl) olive oil

1 garlic clove, minced

lemon juice

herbal salt

pepper (optional)

Instructions

1. Sprinkle the grated cucumber with salt and let sit for 10-15 minutes. In a clean dish towel,

squeeze out as much liquid as you can from the cucumber.
2. Whisk together the yogurt and olive oil until well blended. Add the minced garlic, shredded cucumber and salt. Add a squeeze of lemon to balance the bitterness of the olive oil. Let rest in the refrigerator.
3. Grate the zucchini and follow the same steps as the cucumber to remove the liquid. Mix together with the remaining ingredients and let rest for 5 minutes.
4. Fry the zucchini patties in butter until golden brown on both sides. Serve with broccoli and tomato. on the side.

Prosciutto-Wrapped Salmon Skewers
The fresh flavors of the salmon basil and proscuitto is all you need in this recipe! These flavor dense skewers are a great make ahead item for crowds and buffets.

Ingredients, 8 skewers

Finely-chopped basil

1⅓ lbs (600 g) salmon filet pieces, slightly frozen

1 pinch black pepper

4 slices prosciutto

1 tablespoon olive oil

8 wooden skewers

Instructions

1. Soak the wooden skewers in water to prevent from burning.
2. Finely chop the basil with a sharp knife.
3. Cut the almost thawed salmon pieces length-wise and place onto the skewers.
4. Roll the skewers in the chopped basil and pepper
5. Wrap the prosciutto slices around the salmon.
6. Rub the salmon skewers generously with olive oil and fry in a pan, oven or on the grill.
7. Serve with a hearty salad and a rich aioli or mayonnaise!

TIP! It's easier to thread the salmon onto the skewers when the fish is still slightly frozen.

7. LCHF Snacks and Desserts

While on the LCHF diet, you'll likely notice that you don't need to eat as often. Many people do quite well on two or three meals per day. If you find yourself constantly getting hungry between meals, you're probably not eating enough fat. Don't fear fat! Try increasing your fat intake until you feel satisfied.

Here are quick snack options if you want to eat something right away:

- Rolled-up cheese or ham with a vegetable (some people even spread butter on cheese)
- A piece of cheese
- A hard boiled egg from the refrigerator
- Canned mackerel in tomato sauce
- <u>Babybel cheese</u>

TV Snacks
Olives and nuts are a great replacement for potato chips as TV snacks. Here are more options:
- Mixed nuts
- Sausage: Cut it in pieces, add a piece of cheese and stick a toothpick through them.
- Vegetables with dip, Try cucumber sticks, red, yellow or green peppers, cauliflower, etc.
- Cream cheese rolls: Roll some cream cheese in a piece of salami, air-dried ham or a long slice of cucumber.
- Olives
- LCHF Parmesan chips: On a baking tray, form small piles of grated Parmesan cheese. Heat in oven at 225°C (450°F). Let them melt and get a nice color (be careful, they burn easily). Taste wonderful with dip.

A Delicious LCHF Appetizer – Cheese Puffs
10 pieces
Ingredients
5¼ oz (150 g) soft cheese (preferably a President Brie)
Instructions
1. Dice the brie cheese into cubes, about ½ inch (1×1 cm), removing the rind while doing so. Place the brie cheese cubes on parchment paper

lined plate and heat in the microwave on high for 1–2 minutes. Pay close attention to not burn the cheese pieces.
2. Make a few at the time. Let cool before serving.
Tip:Season with spices of your choice, barbecue seasoning is an excellent choice!

LCHF Pancakes with Berries and Whipped Cream

2 servings

Ingredients
- 4 large eggs
- ½ pound (250 g) cottage cheese
- 2 tablespoons ground psyllium seed husk
- 2 tablespoons butter or coconut oil

Serve with

½–¾ cup (1–2 dl) fresh blueberries, raspberries or strawberries
full fat yogurt or fresh whipped cream

Instructions
1. Whisk together the first three ingredients until well combined. There will still be some lumps, that's OK! Let rest for at least 5 minutes.
2. Heat butter or oil in a frying pan, don't let the cottage-cheese lumps stick to the pan as they melt. Fry the pancakes on medium heat for 3–4 minutes on each side. Flip carefully.

3. Serve with fresh berries and/or whipped cream.

Coconut and Chocolate Mousse à la LCHF
4 servings
Ingredients

    1¾ cups (400 ml) creamy coconut milk

    2 egg yolks

    3½ oz (100 g) dark chocolate (at least 70%)

    1 vanilla stem

Instructions

1. Slowly and carefully bring coconut milk and egg yolks to a simmer, whisking continuously. Let simmer, on low heat, for 10 minutes, stirring often.

2. Roughly chop the dark chocolate and add to a bowl.

3. Carefully split open the vanilla stem with a sharp knife and scrape out the seeds. Add vanilla to the chocolate and pour the hot coconut milk mixture on top. Let stand for about 5 minutes, until the chocolate is melted.

4. Whisk the chocolate mixture together until smooth and creamy and pour into glasses. Refrigerate for at least two hours before serving.

Bacon-Wrapped Halloumi Cheese with Pesto Dip
4 servings

Ingredients

- 1 packet of halloumi cheese
- 1 packet of bacon
- 1 tub of sour cream
- Pesto

Instructions

1. Preheat oven to 450°F (225°C)
2. Slice up a package of halloumi cheese into 8–10 pieces
3. Wrap a piece of bacon around each piece of halloumi and place on a baking sheet.
4. Bake until nicely colored, 10–15 minutes (turning halfway through).

Pesto dip:

Mix a couple of tablespoons of pesto (to taste) with sour cream – done!

Low Carb High Fat Diet & Cookbook

Printed in Great Britain
by Amazon